D0949679

1/4 tps = 1.25 milliliters
1 tps = 5 milliliters
1 tblb = 15 milliliters
1/4 c = 63 ml
1 c = 250 ml.
1/2 gal = 1.9 liters
1 gallon = 3.8 liters

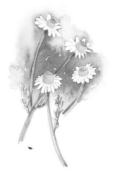

PRACTICAL

A*romatherapy*

PRACTICAL

Aromatherapy

create your own personalized
beauty treatments and natural remedies
using essential oils

Deborah Nixon

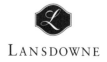

LANSDOWNE

Published by Lansdowne Publishing Pty Ltd
Level 5, 70 George Street, Sydney NSW 2000, Australia

First published in 1995 for Bookmart Limited

Managing Director: Jane Curry
Publishing Manager: Deborah Nixon
Production Manager: Sally Stokes
Project Coordinator/Editor: Bronwyn Hilton
Designer: Michelle Wiener
Cover design: Catherine Martin
Illustrator: Sue Ninham

Set in 9/13pt Bauer Bodini on Quark Xpress
Printed in Singapore by Tien Wah Press (Pte) Ltd.

ISBN 1 86302 417 4

Note: The publishers, author and distributor cannot accept any
responsibility for misadventure resulting from the use of essential oils or
any methods mentioned in this book. No expressed or implied guarantee
can be given nor liability taken.

A note on measurements: For this book measurements are simplified, as
exact conversions are not necessary. The proportion of essential oil to
carrier oil or water is the most important ratio. Just because a little is
beneficial, it does not mean that a large amount will work better. Use only
the recommended proportions and use less for children or if pregnant.

SOME USEFUL CONVERSIONS

3 oz	90–100 mls	5 tablespoons
2 oz	50–60 mls	2 1/2 tablespoons
1 oz	25–30 mls	6 teaspoons (approx. 600 drops)
20 mls	1 tablespoon	
10 mls	2 teaspoons (approx. 200 drops)	
5 mls	1 teaspoon (approx. 100 drops)	
1 ml	20 drops	

4

Contents

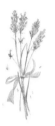

Introduction

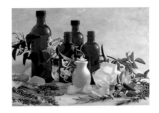

*W*hy this book? There have been many books published on essential oils and aromatherapy in the past decade as the awareness and popularity of essential oils has grown. I am indebted to the many experts and authorities on the subject for having written their books so that I could learn about and experiment with the oils and combinations that suited me.

This book is for those who wish to use essential oils without having to research and study the subject in depth. My aim in writing it was to make it easy for the beginner. So here, in this one small volume, are "recipes" that can be used for all those most common ailments of the mind, body and spirit that are ever present in our fast-paced modern world — from anxiety and aching muscles, hair problems and headaches, to sleeplessness and stress.

The recommendations in this book are not meant to take the place of treatment by a medical practitioner. Before treating any health condition always consult your doctor and a qualified aromatherapist.

One's reactions to smells are highly personal and will change. Experiment with the suggestions in this book until you find the oil or combination of oils that suits you, your health condition, or just your mood for the day. Enjoy!

The Art of Aromatherapy

The pleasure of using the pure essences of fragrant plants has been recognized for centuries. Harness the therapeutic and beneficial properties of oils to enhance every aspect of your health and well-being. You can use essential oils in many ways and most methods do not require any special equipment.

Atomizers (sprays and spritzers)

Use glass, not plastic. Fill with distilled, purified or spring water. If bottled water is not available, use cooled boiled water. Add 3–6 drops of essential oil to each 1 oz (30 mls) of water. Make up only enough for immediate use and re-fill as required. Use to fragrance a room or refresh the face.

Baths

Fill the bath with hand-hot water and then add the essential oils. Disperse the oils well before getting in. Use about 6–12 drops of essential oil for each bath. Alternatively, rub on some blended massage oil before getting into the bath.

Footbaths

Add 4–8 drops of essential oil to a bowl of warm to hot water. Soak for about 15 minutes to refresh the feet.

Sitz baths (hipbaths)

A good method for localized healing. Fill a large plastic bowl with hot or cool to tepid water depending on the treatment required. Add 6–8 drops of essential oil and agitate before immersing the affected area.

Showers

Sprinkle 2 or 3 drops of essential oil onto a damp washcloth and rub over the body while under the shower.

Compresses

Fill a glass bowl with hot or cold water and add 3–12 drops of essential oils. Agitate well to disperse the oils. Place a cotton cloth, washcloth or towel on top of the water; squeeze out and apply to the area to be treated. Use hot compresses for arthritis, neuralgia, muscle ache, back pain, menstrual cramps and skin inflammation. Use cold compresses for headaches, bruises, eye aches and tension. For cramps, colic, swelling, sprains, and bruises, hot or cold compresses can be used. Leave on for about 20 minutes or until the compress reaches body temperature.

Direct application

Not usually recommended. Lavender and tea tree are the exceptions. Apply a dampened cotton bud or sterile cotton gauze cloth sprinkled with a drop of oil to the affected spot.

Inhalation

Fill a glass bowl with very hot, near-boiling water and add 4–10 drops of your chosen essential oils. Place a towel over the head and breathe deeply. Alternatively, sprinkle a drop of essential oil onto a tissue or handkerchief. Use to hydrate, cleanse and stimulate, and for mental fatigue, sinus problems, congestion and colds.

Vaporizers (fragrancers, burners and diffusers)
These containers have a bowl at the top and an opening for a candle at the bottom. Fill the bowl with hot water and add the essential oils. The candle keeps the water heated, releasing the fragrance into the atmosphere. Use 5–15 drops of essential oil. Take care not to let the water evaporate completely as the oils will leave a sticky residue in the bowl.

Massage oils
Add the chosen essential oils to base carrier oils for massage and beauty treatments. Measure 2 oz (50 ml) base oil into a glass bowl or bottle, add 10–25 drops of essential oils and blend. Store in a well-sealed dark glass bottle in a cool dark place, and shake well before each use.

For massage the usual proportion is about 2–3 drops essential oils to 1 teaspoon (5 ml) carrier oil. You need only about a teaspoonful for each massage. Where a stronger blend is indicated for healing, use about 15 drops in 1 oz (30 ml).

Base carrier oils
Because essential oils are very highly concentrated they are best diluted in base carrier oils to enhance their penetration power. Use only 100% pure unrefined cold pressed vegetable, nut or seed oils, not mineral oils.

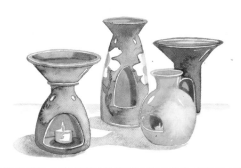

Recommended Base Carrier Oils

Avocado: A nourishing, rich and heavy oil rarely used on its own. Add 10% to other base oils to aid penetration. Good for dry skin conditions.

Evening Primrose: Good for dry skin. Add 10% to other base carrier oils.

Grapeseed: A clear, fine oil with no smell. Excellent for massage.

Hazelnut: Slightly astringent. Good for oily skins. A good penetrative oil.

Jojoba: This is not an oil but a liquid wax and does not turn rancid. Non-greasy and highly penetrative. Use 100% or add to other base oils. Excellent for the face and hair.

Olive: A good basic oil with a strong aroma. Use with other base oils.

Peach or apricot kernel: Good for mature, sensitive or dry facial skin.

Safflower: Good for all skin types.

Sunflower: Good for all skin types.

Sweet almond: An excellent general purpose base oil for all skin types.

Vitamin E: Good for facial use. Mix with sweet almond or jojoba oils to activate penetration of the skin.

Wheatgerm: Anti-oxidant. Too rich and heavy to use on its own. Add 10% to any blend to prevent oxidization and rancidity, and to provide vitamin E. A nourishing oil, good for mature skin and dry skin conditions.

A FACIAL BASE CARRIER OIL BLEND	A BODY MASSAGE BASE CARRIER OIL BLEND
To make 2 oz (50 mls):	**To make 2 oz (50 mls):**
sweet almond 3 tsp (15 mls)	*sweet almond or grapeseed oil 1 1/2 tbsps (30 mls)*
peach kernel 3 tsp (15 mls)	*jojoba oil 1 tsp (5 mls)*
jojoba 3 tsp (15 mls)	*avocado oil 1 tsp (5 mls)*
vitamin E 1 tsp (5 mls)	*wheatgerm oil 1 tsp (5 mls)*

Essential Notes

Essential oils are classified as top, middle and base notes. This is very subjective but generally the top notes are the fastest acting and quickest to evaporate, lasting 3–24 hours. These are the most stimulating and uplifting oils. The middle notes are moderately volatile, lasting 2–3 days, and affect the metabolism and body functions. The base notes are slower to evaporate, lasting up to one week, and are the most sedating and relaxing oils.

Top note oils: basil, bergamot, clary sage, eucalyptus, fennel, grapefruit, lemon, lemongrass, peppermint, rosemary, tea tree

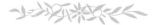

Middle note oils: chamomile, cypress, fennel, geranium, hyssop, juniper, lavender, melissa, orange, petitgrain, pine, rose, tangerine, thyme

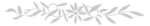

Base note oils: cedarwood, frankincense, jasmine, marjoram, myrrh, neroli, orange, patchouli, sandalwood, ylang ylang

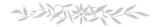

*Use only pure, natural essential oils
from a reputable company. The essential
oils recommended in this book are
the most popular, useful and
readily available essential oils.*

Essential Effects

Basil	uplifting, refreshing, clarifying, aids concentration
Bergamot	refreshing, uplifting
Chamomile	refreshing, relaxing, calming, soothing, balancing
Cedarwood	sedating, calming, soothing, strengthening
Clary sage	warming, relaxing, uplifting, calming, euphoric
Cypress	relaxing, refreshing, astringent
Eucalytpus	head clearing, antiseptic, decongestant, invigorating
Fennel	carminative, eases wind and indigestion
Frankincense	relaxing, rejuvenating, eases breathing, dispels fears
Geranium	refreshing, relaxing, balancing, harmonizing
Hyssop	decongestant
Jasmine	relaxing, soothing, confidence building
Juniper	refreshing, stimulating, relaxing, diuretic
Lavender	refreshing, relaxing, therapeutic, calming, soothing
Lemon	refreshing, stimulating, uplifting, motivating
Lemongrass	toning, refreshing, fortifying
Marjoram	warming, fortifying, sedating
Melissa	uplifting, refreshing
Myrrh	toning, strengthening, rejuvenating, expectorant
Neroli	relaxing, dispels fears
Orange	refreshing, relaxing
Patchouli	relaxing, enhancing to sensuality
Peppermint	cooling, refreshing, head clearing
Petitgrain	refreshing, relaxing
Pine	refreshing, antiseptic, invigorating, stimulating
Rose	relaxing, soothing, sensual, confidence building
Rosemary	invigorating, refreshing, stimulating, clarifying
Sandalwood	relaxing, warming, confidence building, grounding
Tea tree	antiseptic, strengthening to immune system
Thyme	antiseptic, refreshing, strengthening to immune system
Ylang ylang	relaxing, soothing, enhancing to sensuality

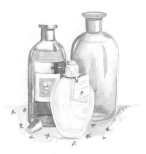

PERSONALIZED
Perfumes

The sense of smell is the most direct trigger of
our emotions. Certain smells inspire
romance, others just make us feel good. There is
nothing nicer than to surround oneself with a
pleasing aroma. Whether your preference is for
the heavy sweet oils or the light and fresh,
experiment until you find a scent that suits you.
You may prefer a lighter perfume on
hot summer days while an exotic heady scent is
perfect for a romantic evening.

The strength of your perfume will depend on the ratio of essential oil to the base oil, alcohol or water. As a general guide, for perfume use a 10% dilution, for eau de toilette use a 5% dilution, for a splash cologne or atomizer spray use a 1% dilution.

If pure alcohol is not available or you do not like the idea of splashing yourself with vodka, jojoba oil makes an ideal base as it will not oxidize and become rancid. For refreshing colognes simply add your chosen essential oils to distilled or spring water and shake vigorously.

A WORD
OF
WARNING:

Too much
perfume can be
overpowering;
err on the side
of caution and
remember, less
is more!

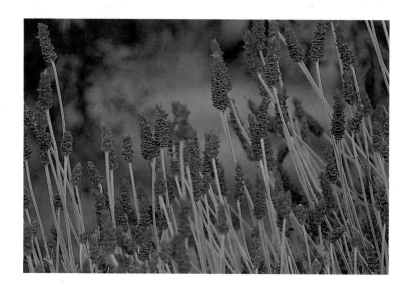

My personal preference is to use 1 or 2 oils only in an atomizer filled with water. For those hot flustered days, a blend of 1–2 drops each of bergamot and lavender or bergamot and geranium makes a refreshing cologne. And there are always those old favorites of rose and lavender.

Begin by mixing together 2 teaspoons (10 mls) jojoba oil and 20 drops (1 ml) essential oil(s) in a dark glass bottle, shake, and keep a few days for the oils to merge. If this is too strong or overpowering for you add more jojoba oil to the mix to make it more subtle.

The following blends can also be used in an atomizer filled with water. Adjust the quantities of the essential oils accordingly.

FLOWERY
*bergamot 8 drops, geranium 8 drops,
neroli 4 drops*

MUSKY
*patchouli 6 drops, sandalwood 4 drops,
ylang ylang 4 drops, rose 4 drops, jasmine 2 drops*

SWEET
*rose 5 drops, rosewood 5 drops, neroli 5 drops,
cedarwood 5 drops*

SPICY
*sandalwood 10 drops, cedarwood 5 drops,
rosewood 4 drops, lemongrass 1 drop*

ROMANTIC
*rose 4 drops, sandalwood 12 drops,
geranium 2 drops, rosewood 2 drops*

The following blends are more subtle. In 2 teaspoons (10 mls) jojoba oil add 2 drops of essential oils. Apply to your wrists, behind your ears, wherever!

CALMING
geranium 1 drop
lavender 1 drop

REFRESHING
geranium 1 drop
orange 1 drop

UPLIFTING
rosewood 1 drop
clary sage 1 drop

EAU DE TOILETTE
bergamot 8 drops
lavender 2 drops
lemon 3 drops
neroli 2 drops
orange 4 drops
rosemary 1 drop

Add to 1 tablespoon (20 mls) distilled water in an atomizer. Shake before use.

If you do not wish to wear a perfume you can still surround yourself with a pleasing fragrance by scenting your clothing and bed linen.

To perfume your lingerie add 1 drop of your chosen essential oil to the final rinse water of the washing. Try rose, geranium, jasmine, neroli or ylang ylang. Take care to ensure the oil is well dispersed in the water and does not touch the lingerie directly.

To give a fresh aroma to towels add 1 drop of lemon in the rinse water or sprinkle a drop in the clothes dryer.

A drop of lavender in the final rinse will impart a lingering restful aroma to sheets and bed linen.

Try a little patchouli or cedarwood on a cotton ball to protect clothes from moths. But use sparingly or the smell could be too heavy.

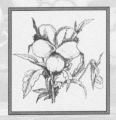

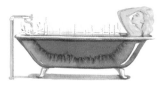

THE

Aromabath

The aromabath is one of the easiest and most
delightful ways to indulge oneself. Whether you wish to
treat a specific health condition or merely rest
and recuperate, the mix of hot water, aromatic oils,
quiet time and privacy is unbeatable.
The therapeutic benefits of an aromabath are twofold:
oils are absorbed through the skin and enter
the circulatory system, and their fragrance is
inhaled through the olfactory system.
Wait until the bath is almost full before adding
the oils, as they evaporate quickly.
The water should be "hand hot", that is as hot as
you can stand but not so hot that you will
feel faint. Avoid very hot water if you are pregnant
or have a heart condition, varicose veins or
broken capillaries.

Relaxation Bath

Use relaxing and calming oils such as bergamot, cedarwood, chamomile, frankincense, lavender, marjoram, neroli, rose, sandalwood, ylang ylang.

Lavender and marjoram are particularly useful if you are having problems sleeping at night. If you are frazzled after a hard day, unwind before bed in a hot bath to prepare for a restful night's sleep. Create a peaceful ambience with candlelight and soft music. Support your head on a bath pillow or rolled up towel, close your eyes and inhale. Concentrate on your breathing and empty your mind of worries. The therapeutic properties of the essential oils will soothe away your stress. After 15-20 minutes, emerge relaxed and wrap yourself in a large, warm towel. Bliss.

Refreshing Bath

Use invigorating and stimulating oils such as cypress, eucalyptus, fennel, geranium, juniper, lemon, lemongrass, peppermint, pine, rosemary, thyme.

Use these oils in the bath for a kick-start in the morning, after a long flight or before an evening out. Keep the bath water tepid and rinse with water as cool as you can bear by adding more cold water to the bath. Rub yourself vigorously with a towel to dry off and splash your face with cool water.

r e c i p e s

Use 6–12 drops of essential oils to a bathtub full of water. If preferred, mix the essential oils with 1 tablespoon (20 mls) of base carrier oil before adding to the bath. Better still, massage yourself with the oil before bathing. Good base carrier oils for aromabaths are sweet almond oil and jojoba oil as they work to nourish and soften the skin.

BURNOUT'S BATH OR THE FRIDAY NIGHT SPECIAL
In a warm bath, add:
lavender 4 drops
geranium 2 drops
neroli 2 drops
Breathe out, lie back, and relax. Guaranteed.

BALANCING
geranium 2 drops
neroli 2 drops
rose 2 drops
If you are feeling at sixes and sevens, this aromatic bath will make you feel more grounded.

CLEANSING AND REFRESHING
lemon 3 drops
geranium 3 drops
I found this blend to be beneficial when travelling in smoggy, polluted cities.

NERVOUSNESS AND OVER-EXCITEMENT
geranium 6 drops
basil or neroli 4 drops
This blend of oils is great for job interviews.

RELAXING
lavender 2 drops
bergamot 2 drops
cedarwood 2 drops
This mix of oils is particularly calming, balancing and uplifting.

RELAXING
frankincense 6 drops
patchouli 4 drops
bergamot 2 drops
This blend is conducive to a meditative state of mind.

RELAXING
chamomile 4 drops
lavender 2 drops
neroli 4 drops
marjoram 2 drops

If insomnia is a problem, a
bath with any combination of
these oils will help ensure a
restful sleep.

RELAXING
lavender 3 drops
clary sage 3 drops

A relaxing blend for
premenstrual tension.

RELAXING
lavender 4 drops
orange 2 drops
cedarwood 2 drops

Try this mix if a stressful
evening is anticipated.

RELAXING
chamomile 3 drops
lavender 3 drops
geranium 2 drops

When a feeling of peace and
harmony is desired.

RELAXING MUSCLES
rosemary 4 drops
marjoram 2 drops
lavender or chamomile 3 drops

Omit the marjoram if feeling
depressed.

RESTORATIVE
lavender 4 drops
geranium 2 drops
clary sage 2 drops

This is a good blend if you are
tired at the end of the day but
need to carry on through
the night.

REVITALIZING
rosemary 3 drops
lemon 2 drops
frankincense 2 drops

This is a great pick-me-up. It is
perfect if you are tired or have
jet lag, are feeling a little
anxious, and need to be alert.

REVITALIZING
rosemary 3 drops
geranium or bergamot 3 drops
Before a night out soak in a
bath to which these oils have
been added.
Add 1 or 2 drops of clary sage if
feeling a little despondent.

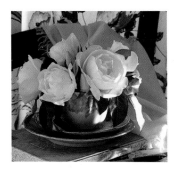

Fragrances

FOR THE HOME & WORKPLACE

$\mathscr{A}$romatic oils can delight the senses, calm the nerves, dispel fears and even, if we believe in the practices of old, banish demons from a building. Essential oils will certainly banish unwanted and unpleasant smells and will create a desired atmosphere for a particular occasion.

In the home, there are many uses for essential oils and the methods of fragrancing a room are diverse. Essential oils used in vaporizers, bowls of water, atomizers, light bulb rings, potpourri and candles will disperse lingering scents into the room. The oils chosen will depend on the effect desired.

ROOM FRESHENER

Place in a vaporizer or into a
bowl of hot water:
bergamot 1 drop
lemon 1 drop
geranium 1 drop
clary sage 1 drop
basil 1 drop
This is a good general all-
purpose room freshener. A
drop or two of just lemon and
bergamot will also freshen
a room.

BATHROOM FRESHENER

For the vaporizer:
lavender or bergamot 6 drops
eucalyptus 1 drop
juniper 1 drop
This blend is refreshing and
disinfecting.

KITCHEN FRESHENER

To eliminate cooking smells, add
to a vaporizer:
lemon 6 drops
orange 6 drops

HOUSEWARMING

Just as aromas create atmosphere
and mood, the aromatic imprint
of your home, especially if it is
an older building, may not suit
you. Make the perfume patterns
your own by sprinkling or
spraying your choice of oils in
each room. Frankincense has been
used for centuries to chase away
memories of previous tenants
and a few drops of lemon and
sandalwood in a vaporizer will
make a new house *your* home.

INSECT REPELLENTS

Use tea tree, eucalyptus,
lemongrass or citronella in a
vaporizer or in candles to keep
flies and mosquitoes away, and
use patchouli and cedarwood for
moths. Add a drop to a cotton ball
and place near stored clothing.

INSECT REPELLENT MASSAGE

Add to 1 oz (30 mls) carrier oil:
eucalyptus 6 drops
peppermint 3 drops
cedarwood 3 drops
Rub onto exposed limbs.

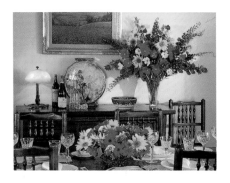

Party Perfumes

*C*reate a party atmosphere with the following oils and oil blends. Use 2–4 drops of each oil in a vaporizer, bowls of hot water, or sprinkle them around the room.

Clary sage will invoke a euphoric feeling. Geranium, lavender, sandalwood and rose will encourage people to unwind and orange is said to promote communication. Bergamot, orange and rosewood are fresh and uplifting oils appropriate for a summer party. A blend of rosewood, bergamot and lavender is also good for setting the mood for a party.

CHILDREN'S PARTY
Orange and lemon are a fresh and joyful combination.

CHRISTMAS
A blend of frankincense and pine will create a celebratory ambience. Other festive oils are myrrh, cedarwood, sandalwood and orange.

ST VALENTINE'S DAY
Ylang ylang and rose are a romantic blend. Sandalwood and patchouli will evoke an exotic atmosphere. For more romantic blends see Sensual Scents, page 66.

Workplace

Studies have been conducted in Japan which show that productivity increased markedly when essential oil of lemon was placed in the air conditioning ducts of factories and offices. This oil promotes motivation and decisiveness. Its refreshing and uplifting qualities also contribute to productivity in the workplace, and being an antiseptic oil it can be used to fight bacteria. When colds and flu are rife, a drop or two of lemon sprinkled around at work can help clear the atmosphere. Combine with other antiseptic oils such as tea tree, bergamot, pine and lavender.

WORKPLACE BLENDS

Use 2 drops of each oil in an atomizer and spray on your face or around the room.

Productivity

Peppermint, lemon and juniper. The peppermint will energize, the lemon motivates and juniper will stimulate and refresh.

Focus

Basil, rosemary and lemon in an atomizer will encourage focus and clarity especially mid afternoon, when energy flags.

Refreshing

Hot and tired? A spray of bergamot in an atomizer will uplift and refresh.

Stress

Balance any mood swings with a water spray of geranium and lavender. To calm yourself try lavender and neroli.

Clear thinking

To stimulate and activate the mind use rosemary and lemon. Rosemary, lemon and basil in a vaporizer will encourage clear thinking.

Any combination of lemon, bergamot, rosemary or rosewood makes a good workplace blend.

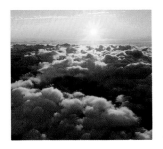

AROMATHERAPY FOR

Mind & Mood

Stress is the scourge of modern life.
We rush from place to place, forget to nurture
ourselves and barely take time for a deep breath.
Add tension, nerves, disappointment, resentment,
anxiety, lack of confidence, grief, lethargy and
fatigue, and it is any wonder we survive at all!

Essential oils with their therapeutic
properties can help to create a calmness of mind
and lightness of mood within all this busyness
and pressure. Aromatherapy is an antidote.
Use these recipes to calm, relax, uplift, balance,
restore and stimulate. The essential oils
will relax and stimulate the nervous system,
enabling the emotional state to be calmed and
leaving you rebalanced and refreshed.

Moods at a glance

Choose one or two oils to alleviate an unwelcome mood or to create the mood you desire.

Angry   chamomile, rose, ylang ylang

Anxious   bergamot, geranium, lavender, neroli, basil

Balance   sandalwood

Concentration   lemon, basil, rosemary

Confidence   frankincense, jasmine, cedarwood, sandalwood, bergamot, neroli, rose

Depression   bergamot, clary sage, patchouli, ylang ylang

Euphoria   clary sage

Fears   frankincense, lavender, sandalwood

Grief   rose, chamomile

Insomnia   bergamot, lavender, marjoram, neroli, orange

Irritability   lavender, neroli, rose, ylang ylang

Memory   basil, rosemary

Nervous butterflies   bergamot, lavender, basil, cedarwood, geranium, neroli

Resentment   rose

Stress   bergamot, lavender, neroli, rose, sandalwood

Mood makers

The constituents of essential oils are closely related to human hormones. Essential oils help rectify adversities caused by hormonal imbalance, providing a form of mood therapy.

Use the following blends in vaporizers, baths, or mixed in 2 oz (50 mls) carrier oil for massages.

Good mood   geranium 5 drops, frankincense 4 drops, neroli or orange 2 drops, jasmine or ylang ylang 2 drops

Euphoric   lavender 2 drops, orange 2 drops, clary sage 6 drops

Grounding   bergamot 3 drops, lavender 3 drops, sandalwood 4 drops

Pampering   rose 4 drops, neroli 2 drops, lavender 4 drops

Balancing   geranium 4 drops, neroli 3 drops, rose 3 drops

Restorative   clary sage 4 drops, rose and lavender 3 drops

Uplifting   bergamot 5 drops, clary sage 5 drops

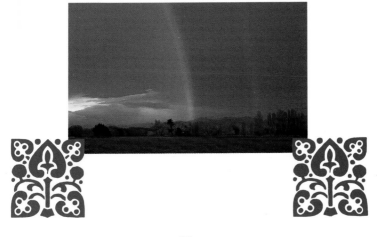

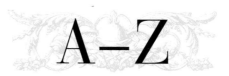

A–Z

of remedies for mind & mood

All these massage blends are for 2 oz (50 mls) base carrier oils.
To use them in an atomizer adjust the quantities accordingly.

ANGER
Bath: chamomile 2 drops, rose or jasmine 2 drops, ylang ylang 2 drops
Bath: geranium 3 drops and rosewood 4 drops
Massage: 20 drops total of rosewood, chamomile, rose or geranium

ANXIETY

Anxiety creates tension in the body and can trigger other stress-related symptoms. Ease your anxiety using the calming and uplifting oils — whether it's an acute bout of nerves or fear, or a long-term problem.

Good oils to use are basil, bergamot, frankincense, rose, geranium, jasmine, lavender, marjoram, neroli, rosewood and sandalwood. See also Nervous tension, page 37.

For nervous butterflies: bergamot 12 drops, basil 5 drops, lavender 8 drops

To calm the nerves: lavender 10 drops, geranium 5 drops, sandalwood 10 drops

For anxiety and depression: 20 drops total of bergamot, neroli, geranium and lavender

For anxiety and fear: lavender 6 drops, frankincense 8 drops, sandalwood 6 drops

To cope with fear: add the grounding, supportive oils such as sandalwood, cedarwood and patchouli to your bath or massage blends.

Daytime bath for anxiety and depression:
clary sage 4 drops, bergamot 2 drops

Night-time bath for anxiety and depression:
lavender 4 drops, jasmine 2 drops, ylang ylang 4 drops

APATHY

Massage: orange 10 drops, frankincense 6 drops, sandalwood 6 drops, and neroli 3 drops. Or sprinkle 4 drops total on a tissue or handkerchief.

CONFIDENCE

To boost confidence, wear a perfume blend made up with jasmine or sprinkle a drop on a tissue and inhale. Make up a massage blend with 20 drops total of jasmine, frankincense and sandalwood.

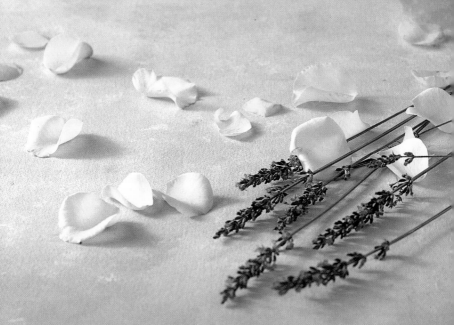

DEPRESSION

Everyone feels low from time to time. Aromatherapy will lift the spirits and could help prevent chronic depression setting in. Geranium, lavender and bergamot are a hard combination to beat. Use in equal quantities in the bath or massage blend. And put a few drops of lavender on your pillow at night.

Uplifting massage: bergamot 10 drops, basil 5 drops, neroli 5 drops and patchouli 5 drops. Or try clary sage 10 drops, neroli 5 drops, sandalwood 5 drops, ylang ylang 5 drops.

Pampering massage: a lovely blend for those "blue" days is rose 10 drops and clary sage 10 drops

Depression defeater massage: rosemary 6 drops, peppermint 6 drops, lemon 3 drops. Use as massage blend or add a spoonful to the bath.

If depressed and sad, ylang ylang, rose or clary sage will give you a boost and if lacking self-esteem and feeling low, a few drops of clary sage and ylang ylang in a bowl of hot water or in a vaporizer during the day will help.

DESPAIR

Massage: sandalwood 10 drops, neroli 10 drops, geranium 5 drops

DISAPPOINTMENT

At times it can seem as though life is full of disappointments and
unfairness. Letting go of resentment and anger and finding a level of
acceptance is instrumental in alleviating or avoiding stress-related illness.
Use comforting oils such as rose, lavender and sandalwood, and the oils
which will promote self-esteem and confidence such as jasmine,
patchouli, marjoram and ylang ylang. Rose will help to release
resentment, and chamomile, rose and ylang ylang will diperse any anger.
Have a bath or massage with these oils and you will feel better instantly.

EMOTIONAL EXHAUSTION

Bath: add 3 drops each of rose and frankincense

Massage: combine or use individually 20 drops total of rose,
geranium, neroli, or frankincense

FATIGUE

Oils for coping with mental fatigue are basil, rosemary, rosewood,
lemongrass, lemon, orange, bergamot, grapefruit, peppermint, juniper
and eucalyptus.

If you really cannot stop to relax and are mentally fatigued, rosemary
will stimulate the memory and concentrate the mind and basil will
promote alertness. Sprinkle a few drops around the room or add to a
vaporizer. Eucalyptus and peppermint are also good revivers and lemon
will refresh and motivate you.

My favorite blend is rosemary 3 drops, basil 3 drops, lemon 4 drops
used in a vaporizer.

If you are fatigued and lacking concentration you could also try the
following combinations in a vaporizer:
1. Peppermint 2 drops, basil 2 drops, lemongrass 2 drops
2. Lemon 2 drops, peppermint 4 drops, bergamot 2 drops
3. Peppermint 4 drops, lemon 4 drops, juniper 2 drops.

Everyone needs support during times of loss. A time of
grieving and consequent healing cannot and should not
be avoided or hurried. Whether the loss is the death of a
loved one, losing a job, or a friend moving away, allow
yourself to grieve and take some time to pamper and
nurture yourself. Sandalwood and cedarwood will help to
reduce disorientation or any overwhelming feelings.
Bath: 3 drops each of neroli, rose and jasmine. Or add
4 drops rose and 5 drops neroli to a teaspoon of jojoba oil
and apply to the skin before you bathe.
Massage: frankincense 6 drops, geranium 5 drops,
bergamot 5 drops, neroli 4 drops

GUILT

Massage: sandalwood 8 drops, neroli 8 drops,
geranium 4 drops

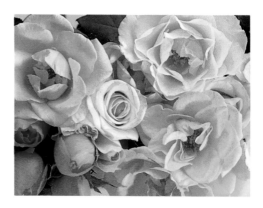

INSOMNIA

Oils to encourage sleep are the calming and sedative oils – lavender, marjoram, neroli and chamomile. Try also cedarwood, orange, geranium, rose and melissa. Create a haven of peace in your bedroom and make it a special place. Place a bowl of dried rose buds in the room and sprinkle them with lavender and rose oils. On the pillows, sprinkle a little lavender, rose, neroli or marjoram.

For a peaceful and relaxed sleep, use the following oils in a vaporizer:

1. Lavender or rose 6 drops
2. Lavender 2 drops and chamomile or cedarwood 4 drops
3. Lavender 4 drops and neroli or bergamot 2 drops
4. Neroli 4 drops and geranium 2 drops
5. Marjoram 5 drops and rosewood 1 drop.

If you wake in the middle of the night, 1–2 drops of marjoram sprinkled on the pillow should help you get back to sleep. Do not use marjoram if you are feeling depressed.

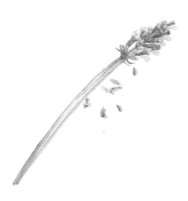

For a peaceful and relaxed sleep, to the bath add:
1. Lavender or neroli 6 drops
2. Chamomile 2 drops, juniper 4 drops, neroli 4 drops
3. Marjoram and rose 2 drops each
4. Lavender 4 drops, marjoram 4 drops, orange 2 drops
5. Lavender 2 drops, chamomile 1 drop, melissa 1 drop
6. Neroli 2 drops, frankincense 2 drops, lavender 2 drops.

   If difficulty in sleeping is caused by emotional distress, add 2 drops each of neroli, lavender and chamomile for a calming and soothing effect.

   If you cannot sleep because of over-excitement, add 3 drops each of marjoram and lavender.

IRRITABILITY

Lavender, geranium, rosewood and rose will soothe the emotions and control irritability. Add 2 drops each to a room vaporizer.

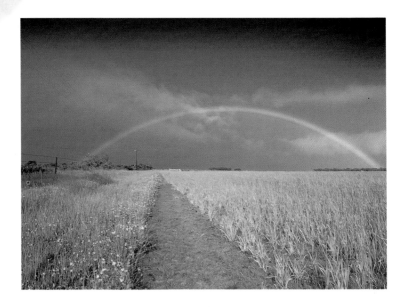

LETHARGY

If suffering from fatigue and inertia, the stimulating oils
— peppermint, cedarwood, bergamot, grapefruit,
eucalyptus, lemon — will give you a jump-start. Add to
the bath, sprinkle on a tissue and inhale, or add to a
room vaporizer.

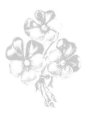

MEMORY LAPSES

Add a drop of rosemary to a tissue and inhale, or place a
cool compress on the forehead and temples. Add 5–6 drops
of rosemary to a bowl of hot water or a vaporizer.

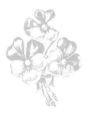

NERVOUS TENSION

Bath: neroli 5 drops; or bergamot 2 drops, marjoram
2 drops, neroli 1 drop, sandalwood 2 drops
Bath: basil 1 drop, juniper 2 drops, lavender 2 drops,
ylang ylang 1 drop
Massage: bergamot 4 drops, marjoram 4 drops, neroli
4 drops, sandalwood 4 drops
Massage: bergamot 10 drops, lavender 12 drops, neroli
8 drops. This is a very calming blend.

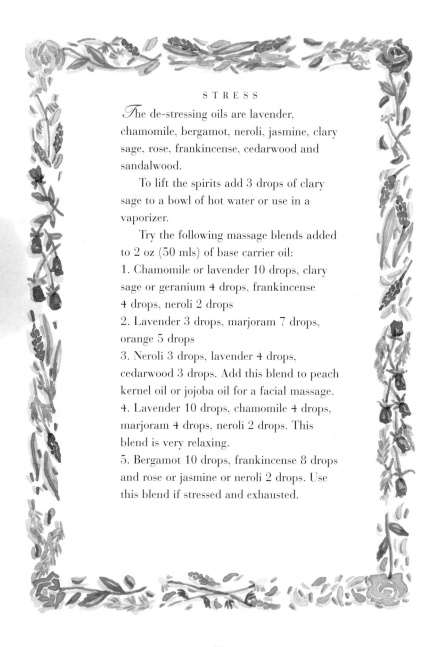

STRESS

*T*he de-stressing oils are lavender, chamomile, bergamot, neroli, jasmine, clary sage, rose, frankincense, cedarwood and sandalwood.

To lift the spirits add 3 drops of clary sage to a bowl of hot water or use in a vaporizer.

Try the following massage blends added to 2 oz (50 mls) of base carrier oil:

1. Chamomile or lavender 10 drops, clary sage or geranium 4 drops, frankincense 4 drops, neroli 2 drops

2. Lavender 3 drops, marjoram 7 drops, orange 5 drops

3. Neroli 3 drops, lavender 4 drops, cedarwood 3 drops. Add this blend to peach kernel oil or jojoba oil for a facial massage.

4. Lavender 10 drops, chamomile 4 drops, marjoram 4 drops, neroli 2 drops. This blend is very relaxing.

5. Bergamot 10 drops, frankincense 8 drops and rose or jasmine or neroli 2 drops. Use this blend if stressed and exhausted.

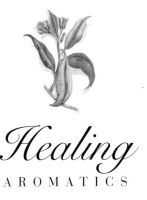

Healing

A R O M A T I C S

Derived from flowers, herbs, trees and fruit,
essential oils have been used for centuries for healing.
In recent times it has been proved that, among other
medicinal qualities, essential oils have antiviral, antiseptic, antibacterial, antifungal and anti-inflammatory
properties. The therapeutic blends in this chapter are
offered as natural tools to assist in the treatment of
physical conditions. They will stimulate the healing and
rejuvination of the mind and body. The following
suggestions are made as an adjunct to supervised medical
treatments. They in no way replace qualified medical
advice. Methods include baths, footbaths, sitz baths,
massage, inhalation and compresses. It is not advised to
apply essential oils directly to the skin or to ingest them
unless supervised by a qualified aromatherapist.
The health conditions listed here are common, treatable
conditions which have responded well to aromatherapy.

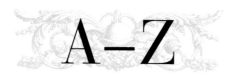

A–Z

of recipes for healing

The massage blends in this chapter are based on approximately 15 drops to every 1 oz (30 mls) of base carrier oil.

ACHING JOINTS/ARTHRITIS

Bath: lavender 2 drops, rosemary 2 drops, marjoram 3 drops
Massage: lavender 5 drops, rosemary 4 drops, marjoram 6 drops

ATHLETE'S FOOT

Footbath: lavender 3 drops, tea tree or eucalyptus 3 drops
Compress: lavender 1 drop, tea tree 1 drop, eucalyptus 1 drop
Massage: tea tree 5 drops, thyme 5 drops, pine 5 drops

BACK PAIN

Massage: rosemary or lemongrass 6 drops, lavender or geranium 6 drops, peppermint 3 drops. This is a stimulating blend. Omit the peppermint for a more relaxing blend.

BLEEDING CUTS AND WOUNDS

Use one of the following essential oils diluted on cotton; apply to affected area: eucalyptus, geranium, lemon, rose or bergamot. Use 1 drop each of lavender and tea tree, diluted on cotton to keep the skin free of bacteria.

BLOOD PRESSURE, HIGH

Caution: Seek your doctor's advice before undertaking any treatment.
Bath: ylang ylang 5 drops, lavender or marjoram 5 drops
Bath: lavender 8–10 drops. The bath should be warm, not hot.
Massage: lavender 8 drops, ylang ylang or neroli 5 drops, marjoram 2 drops

BLOOD PRESSURE, LOW

Bath: sandalwood 3 drops, bergamot 3 drops
Massage: rosemary 7 drops, sandalwood 8 drops, bergamot 5 drops
See also Maternity Mixes, page 69.

BOILS

Apply one drop each of chamomile and lavender diluted on a damp
cotton bud.

BRONCHITIS

Bath or compress: eucalyptus 6 drops, hyssop 2 drops, sandalwood
2 drops
Massage: eucalyptus 7 drops, tea tree 5 drops, lavender 3 drops. Use
half measures for inhalations.

BRUISES

Cold compress: chamomile 1 drop, geranium 1 drop, lavender
1 drop or lavender 2 drops, cypress 1 drop

BRUISES AND SPRAINS

Cold compress: peppermint 3 drops; or lavender and fennel 2 drops
Massage: lavender 6 drops; or lavender 2 drops, chamomile 2 drops,
thyme 2 drops

BURNS

Direct application: lavender 2 drops on a damp cotton bud, or
mix a few drops of lavender in aloe vera gel
Atomizer spray: lavender 10 drops

CATARRH

Massage: eucalyptus 5 drops, cedarwood 3 drops, lemon 5 drops,
pine 5 drops
Inhalation: eucalyptus 2 drops, pine 2 drops, peppermint 2 drops

CELLULITE

Massage: fennel 5 drops, rosemary 4 drops, juniper 2 drops, lavender 4 drops

Massage: cypress 10 drops, rosemary or orange or juniper 5 drops

Bath: cypress 7 drops, rosemary or juniper 3 drops

Bath: juniper 4 drops, orange 4 drops, cypress 2 drops

CHILBLAINS

Warm compress: lemon 3 drops, cypress 3 drops, lavender 3 drops

Massage: lemon 5 drops, cypress 5 drops, lavender 5 drops

Footbath: lavender 4 drops, chamomile 2 drops

COLDS

Bath: lavender 3 drops and rosemary 2 drops — stimulating, for energy

Vaporizer: peppermint 2 drops, eucalyptus 2 drops, rosemary 2 drops, neroli 2 drops

Inhalation: eucalyptus 2 drops, peppermint 2 drops, tea tree 2 drops

Massage for chest infection: tea tree 10 drops — rub on chest

Bath and inhalation for coughs: eucalyptus 4 drops, hyssop 2 drops

Massage for coughs: eucalyptus 5 drops, peppermint 4 drops, basil 3 drops, pine 3 drops

Massage for congestion: lavender 8 drops, eucalyptus 5 drops, juniper 2 drops

Massage to ease breathing: lavender 10 drops or sandalwood 10 drops — rub on chest, neck and throat

Inhalation to ease breathing: eucalyptus, peppermint and pine 2 drops each on a tissue

Head cold bath: basil 4 drops, eucalyptus 4 drops, peppermint 2 drops

Head cold inhalation: basil 4 drops, eucalyptus 4 drops, peppermint 2 drops or 1 drop each on a tissue

Inhalation to remove mucus: bergamot 2 drops, sandalwood 2 drops, eucalyptus 2 drops

CONSTIPATION

Bath: fennel 5 drops, rosemary 5 drops
Massage: lemongrass 5 drops, marjoram 5 drops and rosemary 5 drops. Massage stomach area and lower back.

CRAMPS

Bath: marjoram 5 drops, basil 5 drops
Massage: marjoram 8 drops, basil 7 drops

CYSTITIS

Bath: lavender 3 drops, sandalwood 3 drops, cedarwood 2 drops
Sitz bath: juniper 2 drops, frankincense 2 drops, tea tree 2 drops

DERMATITIS

Bath: geranium 4 drops, juniper 2 drops, lavender 2 drops
Massage: lavender 4 drops, geranium 6 drops, juniper or bergamot 3 drops

DIARRHEA

Massage: 5 drops each of lavender, patchouli, cypress

ECZEMA

Rub: lavender 15 drops in 2 oz (50 mls) aloe vera gel
Compress: bergamot 2 drops, geranium 2 drops, juniper 4 drops, lavender 2 drops
Massage: lavender 10 drops, sandalwood 5 drops
Massage: bergamot 3 drops, geranium 3 drops, juniper 6 drops, lavender 3 drops

EYES

Dilute the oils on a cool damp cotton wool pad. Place on eyes and rest for 10 minutes with eyes closed.

Compress for tired and irritated eyes: chamomile 1 drop
Compress for puffy eyes: chamomile 1 drop
Compress for sore eyes: fennel 1 drop
Cold compress for inflamed or tired eyes: 1 drop of rose or chamomile or lavender

EXHAUSTION

Massage: rosewood 4 drops, neroli 4 drops, geranium 2 drops, lavender 2 drops, jasmine 1 drop, rosemary 2 drops. Use half quantities for a bath.

FEET

Tired feet footbath: rosemary 2 drops, clary sage 2 drops, peppermint 2 drops
Tired and swollen feet footbath: chamomile 3 drops, bergamot 3 drops
Tired, aching feet footbath:
1. Peppermint 2 drops, clary sage 4 drops
2. Juniper or geranium 3 drops, lavender 3 drops, rosemary 3 drops
Tired, aching feet massage: rosemary 9 drops and lavender 6 drops. Use on the whole leg if desired.
Foot smells footbath: cypress 6 drops
Perspiring feet footbath: bergamot 4 drops, clary sage 4 drops, cypress 2 drops
Refreshing footbath: peppermint 3 drops, lemon 3 drops
Better circulation footbath or massage: geranium 2 drops, fennel 2 drops, orange 1 drop

GOUT

Massage: basil 4 drops, rosemary 3 drops, fennel 3 drops, juniper 5 drops. Use half quantities for a footbath.

HANGOVER

Inhalation: rosemary 1 drop or rosewood 1 drop on tissue
Bath: rosemary 3 drops, rosewood 3 drops
Bath: juniper 2 drops, fennel 2 drops and rosemary or basil 1 drop
Cold compress: lavender 1 drop, geranium 1 drop
Cold compress: peppermint 1 drop, rosewood 1 drop, lavender 1 drop
Cold compress: geranium 4 drops, lemon 1 drop
Place the compress over the temples and lie down for 10–15 minutes.
Massage: fennel 6 drops, juniper 2 drops, rosemary or basil 4 drops

HEADACHE

One of the easiest methods to relieve a headache is to apply a damp
tissue or cloth sprinkled with lavender to the temples or to sprinkle one
or two drops of lavender on the edge of your pillow.
Massage: melissa 3 drops or lavender 3 drops on forehead and temples
Cold compress or inhalation: rosemary 1 drop, peppermint
1 drop, chamomile 1 drop, neroli 1 drop. Place compress over forehead
and temples.
Inhalation: rose 1 drop, basil 1 drop, orange 1 drop, rosemary 1 drop
Vaporizer: melissa 4 drops, peppermint 2 drops or chamomile 2 drops
Rub: lavender 1–2 drops neat on neck, temples, forehead, base of skull
Tension headaches
Inhalation: lavender 2 drops, chamomile 1 drop on tissue
Bath: lavender 3 drops, chamomile 3 drops, geranium 3 drops
Massage: lavender 5 drops, chamomile 5 drops, geranium 5 drops

HEARTBURN/INDIGESTION

See Indigestion p.46 and also Maternity Mixes, page 71.

HIVES

Massage: chamomile 4 drops, melissa 4 drops
Compress: chamomile 3 drops, melissa 3 drops
Bath: chamomile 3 drops, melissa 3 drops in a tepid to warm bath.

IMMUNE SYSTEM

Bath: bergamot 2 drops, rosemary 2 drops, eucalyptus 2 drops, geranium 2 drops, tea tree 2 drops

Massage: bergamot 5 drops, lavender 4 drops, eucalyptus 2 drops, tea tree 2 drops. Massage around the kidney area.

INDIGESTION/HEARTBURN

See also Maternity Mixes, page 71.

Compress: peppermint 4 drops or lavender 4 drops. Place on stomach.

Vaporizer: lavender 5–10 drops

Massage: peppermint 2 drops, basil 1 drop, fennel 1 drop, chamomile 1 drop, lavender 1 drop. Massage on stomach and chest.

Massage: basil 3 drops, fennel 5 drops, peppermint 7 drops

INFECTIONS

Add a few drops of tea tree to a cool compress and apply to the infected area.

INFLUENZA

Bath: tea tree 3 drops, lavender 3 drops, eucalyptus 3 drops

Bath: Add 3–4 drops of one oil to the bath: lavender, eucalyptus, sandalwood, tea tree or lemon.

Vaporizer or inhalation: tea tree 2 drops, lavender 2 drops, eucalyptus 2 drops

Massage: lavender 8–10 drops. See also Colds, page 42.

LARYNGITIS

Massage: lavender 5 drops, chamomile 4 drops and tea tree 4 drops. Massage on throat and chest.

MENSTRUATION

Menstrual cramps

Hot compress: clary sage 3 drops, marjoram 2 drops. Place on stomach and lower back.

Massage: sandalwood 5 drops, frankincense 5 drops, orange 5 drops

Massage: clary sage 10 drops; or clary sage 5 drops, chamomile 2 drops, geranium 2 drops, rose 1 drop

Premenstrual tension

Oils for alleviating the symptoms of premenstrual tension are clary sage, rose and geranium. Lavender, ylang ylang and lemongrass are also useful at this time. Clary sage is a hormone regulator.

Bath: geranium 3 drops, clary sage 4 drops, rose 3 drops

Bath: lavender 4 drops, ylang ylang 2 drops, if tense and irritable.

Massage: clary sage 6 drops, geranium or lavender 6 drops and rose 3 drops. Massage the lower back, abdomen and thighs.

Massage: basil 7 drops, geranium 5 drops, rose 3 drops. This is a balancing massage blend.

For water retention and bloatedness: Use fennel, juniper, rosemary, or geranium.

For mood swings, depression and irritability: Use clary sage, bergamot, jasmine, or rose. If feeling ungrounded and emotionally unstable use lemongrass. To calm yourself, rub a little rose mixed in jojoba oil on your wrists or sprinkle on a tissue and inhale.

MIGRAINE

Bath: lavender 2 drops, marjoram 2 drops, melissa 4 drops, sage 2 drops

Compress: lavender 2 drops, marjoram 2 drops, melissa 4 drops, sage 2 drops

Massage: Mix 1 drop each of basil and peppermint in a teaspoon of jojoba oil and rub on each temple.

Inhalation: basil 1 drop, marjoram 1 drop, peppermint 1 drop. Place on a tissue and inhale. See also Headache, page 45.

MUSCULAR PAIN

Hot compress: chamomile 2 drops, rosemary 2 drops, sandalwood 1 drop
Massage: juniper 5 drops, lavender 4 drops, rosemary 4 drops
Bath: eucalyptus 4 drops, rosemary 4 drops
Compress and footbath: eucalyptus 3 drops, rosemary 3 drops

NAUSEA

Vaporizer: peppermint 4 drops
Inhalation: lavender 1 drop, peppermint 1 drop. See also Maternity Mixes, page 71.

NERVE PAIN

For sciatica and neuralgia, use the analgesic oils chamomile, peppermint, lavender, and rosemary. Combine 2 or 3 drops of these oils on a warm compress and apply to the affected area. Place a hot water bottle on top and relax.
Bath: lavender 3 drops, chamomile 3 drops

OEDEMA/SWOLLEN FEET

Massage: lavender 6 drops; or rosemary 3 drops, geranium 3 drops. Rest with legs elevated higher than the head. See also Maternity Mixes, page 71.

PILES/HAEMORRHOIDS

Sitz bath: cypress 8 drops; or cypress 4 drops, geranium or lavender 4 drops. Soak the affected area for 10 minutes or use a compress. Use warm water in the sitz bath.

Compress: patchouli 1 drop, myrrh 3 drops, cypress 2 drops. Juniper and frankincense are also useful in compresses.

Bath: cypress 5 drops, juniper 3 drops, frankincense 3 drops

Massage: cypress 7 drops, lavender or geranium 8 drops.

Or add 15 drops of the essential oils to 2 oz (50 mls) aloe vera gel or a lubricating jelly and rub around area to alleviate the symptoms.

SKIN CONDITIONS

See also Skin types, page 52.

Eczema, dermatitis, psoriasis

Massage: lavender 8 drops, chamomile 3 drops, melissa 3 drops

Massage: bergamot 5 drops, lavender 5 drops, geranium 3 drops

Rashes

Bath: lavender 4 drops, chamomile 4 drops. The water should be warm, not hot.

Cool compress: lavender 2 drops, chamomile 2 drops

Massage: chamomile 3 drops, lavender 8 drops, tea tree 4 drops

Scars

Blend together neroli with lavender or bergamot or chamomile or frankincense into wheatgerm oil and apply to the scar.

SINUS

Vaporizer: Total of 6 drops of eucalyptus, basil, peppermint, thyme, or tea tree. To deepen breathing: frankincense 4 drops

Inhalation: lavender 2 drops, eucalyptus 2 drops

Inhalation: peppermint 2 drops, tea tree 2 drops, eucalyptus 2 drops

Inhalation: eucalyptus 2 drops on a tissue

Bath or massage: basil 2 drops, eucalyptus 3 drops, lavender 2 drops, peppermint 3 drops

Massage: rosemary 2 drops, geranium 2 drops, chamomile 2 drops, eucalyptus 2 drops. Massage nose, forehead, cheeks, ears and neck.

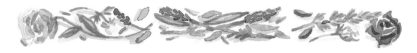

SUNBURN

Lavender and tea tree oils will soothe and heal sunburn. Dilute 2 drops in 3 oz (100 mls) of water (not oil) and spray on, or soak a cold cotton compress or handkerchief in the mix to cool the burn. Lavender added to aloe vera gel is also soothing.

Bath: peppermint 6 drops, lavender 4 drops

THROAT INFECTIONS

Gargle with a drop of tea tree or bergamot added to water.

Sore throat massage: sandalwood 6 drops and clary sage or tea tree 6 drops. Massage the throat and neck, or try 3 drops each of tea tree, sandalwood and clary sage.

TONSILLITIS

Oils for the relief of tonsillitis symptoms are lavender, tea tree, lemon and chamomile. Choose one oil, dilute 1 drop in a glass of water and gargle.

Massage: lavender 6 drops, tea tree 8 drops, lemon 1 drop. Rub on the upper stomach and back.

Compress: lavender 1 drop, tea tree 1 drop, lemon 1 drop, chamomile 1 drop. Use warm water for the compress and place on the throat.

Vaporizer: lavender 1 drop, tea tree 1 drop, lemon 1 drop, chamomile 1 drop

VARICOSE VEINS

Massage: rosemary 5 drops, juniper 5 drops, lemon 2 drops
Bath or massage: cypress 5 drops, geranium 5 drops

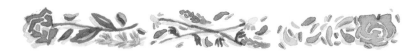

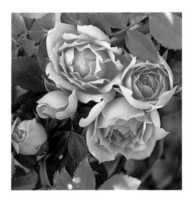

NATURAL
Beauty

The ingredients of good health and beauty
are good food, adequate sleep, an alert mind, plenty of
rest and relaxation, and sensible exercise.
While looking good begins with one's inner health, a
glowing blemish-free skin, shiny hair and
lustrous nails can be helped along with aromatherapy.
Essential oils will moisturize and nourish
the skin, smooth out wrinkles, regenerate skin cells,
stimulate tired skin and help heal inflamed or
infected skin conditions such as pimples and acne.
Choose from the beauty recipes
on the following pages for your skin and hair type.

Skin types and conditions

Choose from the following oils for your skin type.

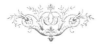

Acne: bergamot, lavender, camphor, geranium, juniper, chamomile, rose, neroli, sandalwood, tea tree, ylang ylang, lemon. The cleansing and antibacterial oils work as natural antiseptics and regulate secretion of sebum.

Chapped skin: chamomile, geranium, lavender, patchouli, rose, sandalwood

Dry skin: cedarwood, geranium, jasmine, lavender, orange, rose, rosewood, ylang ylang, patchouli, sandalwood, chamomile

Inflamed or irritated skin: chamomile, geranium, hyssop, myrrh, peppermint, rose, sandalwood, tea tree, lavender

Itchy skin: cedarwood, jasmine, peppermint, chamomile

Mature skin (for skin rejuvenation and cell regeneration): frankincense, lavender, neroli, rose, sandalwood

Normal skin: bergamot, cedarwood, geranium, lavender, neroli, chamomile, rose, rosewood, sandalwood

Oily skin: bergamot, cedarwood, cypress, frankincense, geranium, juniper, rose; and for pimples: lavender, lemon, tea tree, eucalyptus

Sensitive skin: jasmine, orange, chamomile, rose. Avoid or use sparingly: cedarwood, eucalyptus, lemon, lemongrass, melissa, peppermint, pine, rosemary, thyme

Body massage blends
for good health and beautiful skin

*W*hether giving yourself a massage or enlisting someone's help, choose
the essential oils that are right for your skin type from the following
blends. You do not need to be an expert; the oils will do their work
regardless, and the sheer indulgence will nourish your mind, body and
spirit — a sure path to natural beauty. Experiment with the movements
and amount of pressure that are right for you.

For these blends use 2 oz (50mls) of base carrier oil.

Stimulating: rosewood 8 drops, geranium 4 drops, orange 3 drops

Relaxing: lavender 8 drops, sandalwood 5 drops, melissa 2 drops

Regenerating and stregthening: frankincense 6 drops, geranium
6 drops, cedarwood 3 drops

To strengthen the immune system: lavender 10 drops,
bergamot 5 drops

Before exercise to warm the muscles: rosemary 8 drops,
lavender 7 drops

**After exercise to eliminate toxins and prevent
stiffness:** lavender 8 drops, petitgrain 3 drops, lemongrass 2 drops,
juniper 2 drops. Also use this blend in the bath.

Thigh massage: juniper 6 drops, cypress 6 drops, lavender 3 drops.
Use with jojoba oil.

Dry skin: sandalwood 10 drops, geranium 3 drops, rose 2 drops

Normal skin: lavender 6 drops, sandalwood 4 drops, ylang ylang
3 drops, geranium 2 drops

Oily skin: lemon 7 drops, tea tree 3 drops, cypress 5 drops

Mature skin: lavender 8 drops, frankincense 5 drops, neroli 2 drops

Sensitive skin: rosewood 5 drops, neroli 5 drops, rose or jasmine
5 drops

Facial massage

$\mathcal{A}$ facial massage is sheer bliss. Enhance the experience with your own special blend of essential oils added to a base carrier oil. After cleansing, smooth the oil mix over the face and throat avoiding the eye area. Cover the area by stroking upwards and outwards and continue with circular movements. Do not be too concerned about doing it "right"; whatever feels good will be beneficial.

Some methods to try are: small circular movements with your thumbs; tapping under your chin; pressing your fingertips around the cheekbones and eyebones; applying the fingers to the pressure points above the nose and underneath the eyebrows; smoothing your fingers or palms across the top of the forehead and out to the ears; applying slight pressure with the fingers at either side of the temples. As a general rule keep the movements upwards and outwards, smoothing any tension out and away.

For a facial massage use peach kernel oil, sweet almond oil or jojoba oil. To 1 teaspoon (5 mls) base oil add 1–3 drops essential oil.

Oils for facial massage
Normal skin: bergamot, lavender, sandalwood
Oily skin: basil, cypress, lemon
Dry or mature skin: lavender, geranium, frankincense

Hot compresses

$\mathcal{C}$ompresses are particularly useful if carrier oils are not on hand, or if your skin is oily or sensitive and irritated and you prefer not to use carrier oils. A compress will revitalize and refresh your skin.

Dry skin: rose 2 drops, neroli 1 drop, chamomile 1 drop
Oily skin: rose 1 drop, sandalwood 1 drop, geranium 1 drop
Pimples/acne: lavender 2 drops, lemon 1 drop
Irritated or sensitive skin: chamomile 2 drops, rose 1 drop

Facial steaming

$\mathcal{S}$teaming helps to hydrate, cleanse and stimulate facial skin. Add 5–6 drops of essential oils to a bowl of hot water and wrap a towel around your head to prevent the steam from escaping. Steam for about 5 minutes. Use singly or combined:

Normal skin: bergamot, geranium
Oily skin: lemon, cypress, juniper
Dry or mature skin: geranium, lavender, patchouli, rose
Irritated skin: chamomile, fennel

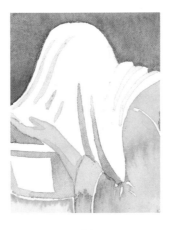

Facial masks

𝒰se clay, ground oatmeal, or a clay base powder such
as "Fuller's Earth". Add hot distilled water and blend
into a paste. Add your chosen essential oils and blend
well. Use 3 drops of essential oils to one teaspoon of base
powder or 15 drops per cup of paste. Smooth the mix
onto a cleansed face, avoiding the skin around the eyes,
leave it to dry (about 10–15 minutes) and then wash off
with tepid water. For a smoother consistency add plain
yoghurt and for very dry or sensitive skin add some
jojoba, sweet almond or vitamin E oil. For dry skin
apply once a week; for oily skin, twice weekly.

OILS FOR FACIAL MASKS

Dry and mature skin: lavender, frankincense,
geranium

Oily skin: cypress, bergamot, juniper

Normal skin: geranium, lavender, eucalyptus

Acne: cypress, lemon, tea tree

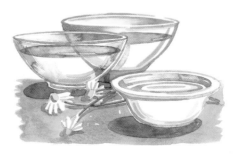

Facial cleansers

$\mathcal{B}$lend your chosen essential oils with a mild, unperfumed brand of cleanser or lotion. Choose the essential oils for your skin type from the list of suitable oils for facial toners.

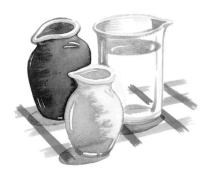

Facial toners

$\mathcal{A}$dd a few drops of your chosen essential oils to an atomizer filled with distilled water for a refreshing toner spritzer. A handy purse-sized atomizer contains 1 oz (30 ml) of water. Always use a glass atomizer and shake well to disperse the oils. For a refreshing facial spray try clary sage for daytime and lavender at night.

OILS FOR FACIAL TONERS

Dry or sensitive skin: rose, sandalwood, chamomile
Dry and normal skin: lavender, geranium, rose, chamomile
Oily skin: bergamot, lavender, juniper, lemon, lemongrass
Acne: bergamot, lavender

Facial moisturizers

The penetrative qualities of essential oils make them ideal nourishing treatments to soften the skin and make it supple and smooth. They will not clog up the pores and will help balance oily and inflamed skin. If you prefer not to use base carrier oils as facial moisturizers, add a few drops of the essential oils for your skin type to a mild, unperfumed brand of moisturizing cream or lotion that contains mostly natural ingredients and not too many preservatives, dyes and chemicals.

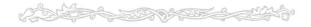

Add the following blends to 2 oz (50 mls) of chosen carrier oils.

Dry skin: sandalwood 6 drops, geranium 4 drops, rosewood 2 drops, ylang ylang 3 drops

Normal to dry skin: geranium 1 drop, lavender 6 drops, sandalwood 4 drops, ylang ylang 4 drops

Normal skin: lavender 8 drops, geranium 5 drops, rose 2 drops

Mature skin: lavender 8 drops, frankincense or sandalwood 3 drops, neroli 2 drops, rose 2 drops

Wrinkles: fennel 8 drops, lavender 2 drops, rose 3 drops

Acne: Add to witch hazel if preferred:
1. Tea tree 15 drops; or tea tree or lemon 7 drops, juniper 3 drops, cypress 3 drops, bergamot 2 drops
2. Lavender or chamomile 15 drops will aid healing, reduce inflammation and prevent scarring.

Oily skin: lemon 6 drops, cypress 5 drops, lavender 4 drops

Irritated skin: sandalwood 5 drops, chamomile 5 drops, rose 5 drops

Hand care

*W*e often neglect our hands, yet they are the first part of the body to show signs of age. Pamper them by soaking in a bowl of warm water with a few drops of lavender added. Dry them gently, then apply a blend of essential oils in a carrier oil and massage.

Essential oils for the hands: lavender, lemon, chamomile, rose, and orange. If sensitive skin: chamomile and melissa.

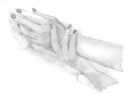

EXFOLIATION

Once a week or for a treat, exfoliate the skin on your hands with the following blend. Follow with moisturizing cream and sunscreen.

Mix together in a glass bowl:

2 tbsps raw sugar

1 tbsp (20 mls) base carrier oil

lavender 2 drops

lemon 2 drops

HAND MASSAGE

Add to 1 oz (30 mls) base carrier oil:

Normal skin: lavender 7 drops, sandalwood 4 drops, geranium 4 drops

Dry skin: patchouli 5 drops, bergamot 8 drops, frankincense 2 drops

Chapped hands: lemon 3 drops, myrrh 4 drops, rose 4 drops, sandalwood 4 drops

NAIL CARE

To strengthen the nails: add lemon 3 drops, rosemary 2 drops, lemongrass 3 drops, lavender 2 drops to 1 oz (30 mls) sweet almond oil and rub into and around the nails. Cypress, lavender and sandalwood are also good for the nails.

Hair essentials

*L*ike your skin and eyes, your hair is a mirror of your health. Keep your hair in good condition with the help of suitable essential oils for the hair: cedarwood, clary sage, cypress, juniper, lavender, lemon, chamomile, rosemary or rosewood. Choose from these for your hair type.

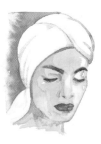

HAIR SHAMPOO

To 15 oz (500 mls) of a natural, mild, unperfumed, non-detergent brand of shampoo or to shavings of pure soap immersed in a bottle of water, add 10 drops essential oils.

> **Dry hair:** cedarwood 10 drops
> **Normal hair:** lavender 10 drops
> or chamomile 10 drops
> **Oily hair:** rosemary 10 drops
> **Hair loss:** cedarwood 5 drops,
> rosemary 5 drops
> **Dandruff:** rosemary 5 drops
> and cedarwood 5 drops, or
> rosemary 10 drops

HAIR RINSES

Hair rinses will impart lustre and shine to your hair.
Choose the essential oils appropriate to your hair type.
Add 4–10 drops of essential oils to 15 fl oz (500 mls)
water in a glass bottle. Shake well and use as a final rinse
after shampooing. Use any favorite oil to surround
yourself with the aroma. For an uplifting effect try
geranium, bergamot or clary sage, and for special
occasions use rose.

Oily hair: cedarwood, cypress,
juniper, lavender, 1 drop each
Dry hair: sandalwood 4 drops
Dandruff: clary sage 2 drops,
lavender 2 drops
Dark hair: rosemary 2 drops,
rosewood or sandalwood 1 drop,
geranium 1 drop
Fair hair: chamomile 2 drops,
lemon 1 drop
White hair (to brighten):
chamomile 4 drops

HAIR CONDITIONER

For extra shiny hair add a chosen essential oil to jojoba
oil and massage through from the roots to the ends of the
hair, or use 10% jojoba and 90% sweet almond oil.

Try rosewood, sandalwood, rose or clary sage, or any
one of the essential oils suitable for your hair type.

Hair treatments

To improve your hair's texture and replace nutrients try a warm oil treatment. Apply once a week to treat damaged hair or pamper yourself monthly. Jojoba oil is an excellent base carrier oil for hair treatments.

Make up a blend of 10–25 drops of essential oils to 2–3 oz (50–100 mls) of base carrier oil depending on the length of your hair. Part the hair into sections. Apply the mixture along the sections all the way down to the ends with hands or cotton wool dipped in the oil. Wrap in a warm towel and leave on for 2 hours for best effect. If possible sit in the sunshine or in a steamy bath. To remove, work in some shampoo and a small amount of water, then wash as normal.

Damaged hair
geranium 5 drops
sandalwood 10 drops
lavender 10 drops

Normal hair
lavender 10 drops
cedarwood or rosewood
20 drops

Dry hair
rosewood 15 drops
sandalwood 10 drops

Oily hair
bergamot 12 drops
lavender 13 drops or try
tea tree 6 drops
lemon 6 drops
geranium 4 drops
lavender 4 drops
This is an antibacterial massage for the scalp.

Thinning hair
lavender 10 drops
rosemary 10 drops
A blend to stimulate and encourage new hair growth.

For dandruff
eucalyptus 10 drops
rosemary 15 drops
Try also
tea tree 25 drops, or
patchouli 10 drops
tea tree 15 drops

To strengthen the hair
rosemary 8 drops
lavender 8 drops
bergamot 4 drops

For dry, itchy scalp
cedarwood and lavender
10 drops each
Bergamot is also beneficial for an itchy scalp.

Sensual Scents

TO ENHANCE YOUR
LOVE LIFE

The sense of smell is central
to our sensuality and the power of scent to inspire
romance has been recorded for centuries.
There is no guarantee that these blends will work
on an unwilling partner, but they will help
create a romantic mood and a calming and sensual
atmosphere. The rest is up to you.

The aphrodisiac oils

Clary sage
sweet and uplifting, euphoric

Geranium
floral, relaxing and uplifting

Jasmine
heady and luxurious

Neroli
dispels anxiety and shyness

Orange
for joy, sensual and soothing

Patchouli
exotic and heady, sensual

Rose
romantic, heady, euphoric

Sandalwood
exotic and spicy

Ylang ylang
relaxing and soothing

*B*eware of combining too many oils together as they may clash and become overpowering. Subtlety is the key.

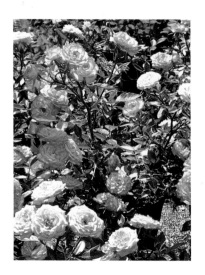

Sensual massage blends

To 2 oz (50 mls) base oil add:

rosewood 13 drops
ylang ylang 8 drops
jasmine 4 drops

jasmine 4 drops
rose 5 drops
sandalwood 10 drops
bergamot 5 drops

rose 5 drops
sandalwood 10 drops
patchouli 5 drops
clary sage 5 drops

Sensual aromabaths

Luxuriate alone and prepare yourself for romance or share an aromabath with your partner.

ylang ylang 4 drops
sandalwood 2 drops

ylang ylang 2 drops
patchouli 2 drops
orange 4 drops

jasmine 4 drops
bergamot 2 drops

sandalwood 4 drops
lavender 2 drops
ylang ylang 2 drops

rose 2 drops
patchouli 2 drops
ylang ylang 2 drops

Body lotions

Pamper your body and enhance your appeal with these blends. Add to 2 oz (50 mls) base oil:
sandalwood 5 drops
jasmine 2 drops
ylang ylang 4 drops
rose 4 drops

ylang ylang 5 drops
patchouli 5 drops
rose 5 drops

Intimate perfumes

Choose from jasmine, ylang ylang, sandalwood and patchouli. Add 2-3 drops to a teaspoon of jojoba oil and use as a perfume. Apply to the pulse points.

Room Fragrances

*C*reate a space for intimacy and romance
by preparing a room with these blends. Use in a vaporizer
or sprinkle around the room.

EXOTIC

patchouli 5 drops
sandalwood 2 drops
rose 2 drops

INTIMATE

sandalwood 5 drops
jasmine 2 drops

WARM

ylang ylang 5 drops
neroli 2 drops
bergamot 1 drop

ROMANTIC

jasmine 3 drops
rose 3 drops

HEADY

rose 2 drops
patchouli 2 drops
jasmine 1 drop
ylang ylang 1 drop

To encourage and enhance a
romantic mood and excite the
senses, combine 1 or 2 drops
each of 2 or 3 of these
essential oils in a vaporizer:
*ylang ylang, jasmine,
sandalwood, patchouli, rose,
clary sage.*

To relax the mind and feel
euphoric, choose from
*clary sage, neroli, patchouli,
rose, ylang ylang.*

Do remember to co-ordinate
these oils with your massage
blends, perfumes and
bath blends.

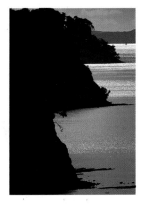

Travel

E S S E N T I A L S

$\mathcal{A}$ few essential oils can make
the difference between a tiring, stressful journey
that leaves you fraught and an enjoyable trip.
To avoid or alleviate the worst symptoms of jet lag
take at least lavender, rosemary, sandalwood,
bergamot and geranium with you.

Flying

On the plane: sprinkle 2 drops lavender and 1 drop ylang ylang on a hot wash cloth and wipe the face and neck.

For anxiety: lavender and geranium on a tissue; inhale.

Swollen feet compress: lavender 5 drops on a damp handkerchief, apply directly

Direct application: lavender 2 drops, ylang ylang 1 drop, on a hot washcloth, apply to face and neck. Sprinkle a drop of lavender on a tissue and rub over pulse points after eating to soothe, calm and promote sleep.

On arrival

If you can, wait until local night-time before preparing for bed, then take a bath with lavender and geranium, or chamomile and lavender, or lavender and marjoram, to assist sleep. A lavender and ylang ylang bath is especially good for night-time arrivals. If bathing in the daytime, rosemary and sandalwood will keep you alert. The next morning, bathe with rosemary and geranium or basil, or peppermint and eucalyptus. If there is no bath, sprinkle the oils onto a wash cloth and massage the body in the shower.

To increase vitality: bath with rosemary and geranium.

To let go of stress and tension: inhale jasmine, lemon or bergamot sprinkled on a tissue.

To sleep: marjoram sprinkled onto tissue or in a vaporizer, or bath with lavender.

Travel sickness: inhale peppermint on a tissue

Travel fatigue: massage neck with lavender

For hotel rooms

Fill a bowl or ashtray with hot water and add a drop of tea tree, lemon, eucalyptus or rose, to freshen the room.

Maternity

MIXES

Pregnancy is a time of physical and emotional change
and essential oils can play a part in dealing
with the stresses of pregnancy and labor and with
postnatal recuperation as well as enhancing the joys
of this very special time. Some essential oils should be
avoided during pregnancy and others should not
be used during the first three or four months (see below).
Be cautious; use low doses and consult a qualified
aromatherapist. During my own pregnancy I used
lavender, neroli, frankincense, sandalwood, geranium,
lemon and rose most frequently.

Recommended oils

lavender, tangerine, chamomile, frankincense, rose,
neroli, sandalwood, geranium, lemon and rose
Use in vaporizers, in massage, or just sprinkled
on a tissue or around the room.

Oils to avoid

anise, basil, camphor, caraway, carrot,
cedarwood, cinnamon, clary sage, clove, cypress, fennel,
hyssop, jasmine, juniper, marjoram, mint, myrrh,
nutmeg, oregano, pennyroyal, rosemary, sage,
sassafrass and thyme
Avoid in first three months: chamomile,
frankincense, geranium, melissa, and rose

Special aromabath blends
for pregnancy

(Baths taken during pregnancy should be warm, not hot.)
Refreshing: bergamot 3 drops, rosewood 3 drops. This
is a good blend for the hot summer months.
Other light, refreshing oils are lemon, orange and neroli.

Relaxing: lavender 3 drops, geranium 3 drops

Soothing: neroli 3 drops, rose 2 drops, ylang ylang
1 drop. See also The Aromabath (page 19).

Special massage blends
for pregnancy

These blends are for 2 oz (50 mls) of base carrier oil.
Indulgence: lavender 5 drops, rose 5 drops,
frankincense 5 drops. This luxurious blend is perfect for
the later months; lavender will relax you, frankincense
will dispel any anxiety and rose will pamper you.

Morale booster: geranium 15 drops

Relaxation: neroli 5 drops, frankincense 5 drops,
sandalwood 5 drops

Abdomen: lavender or neroli 15 drops

Legs and feet: geranium 7 drops, lavender 8 drops

Lower back: bergamot 8 drops, geranium 3 drops,
sandalwood 4 drops

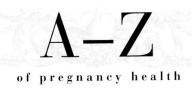

A–Z

of pregnancy health

Refer also to Healing Aromatics, page 39 and
Aromatherapy for Mind & Mood, page 27.

Braxton Hicks contractions: sprinkle lavender on your pillow or
add to a warm bath

Heartburn/indigestion: Peppermint is helpful for heartburn and
indigestion but use in very low dosages. Add 1 drop to 1 tablespoon (20 mls)
of base oil and rub on chest and upper stomach. Sandalwood is also good.
Avoid rich, heavy meals. Try a drop of lemon or lavender in a vaporizer.

High blood pressure massage: neroli 5 drops, lavender 5 drops
and rose or ylang ylang 5 drops in 2 oz (50 mls) base oil.

Morning sickness/nausea: try 1 drop of lemon in a vaporizer, and
1 drop of lavender in a cool compress applied to the stomach. Inhale a
little peppermint diluted on a tissue.

Oedema/swollen feet massage: lavender 8 drops, geranium
7 drops in 2 oz (50 mls) base oil. Try a cool compress with lavender. Lie
down for at least 10 minutes every day with the feet elevated.

Stretch marks: a gentle daily massage on the stomach and hips will
help keep the skin supple. Try lavender 10 drops and neroli 5 drops in
2 oz (50 mls) wheatgerm oil, evening primrose oil or vitamin E oil. As
vitamin E oil is hard to rub in, mix it with jojoba and sweet almond oil
for easier application and penetration. Try also lavender, neroli and rose;
or lavender, rose and frankincense.

The birthing room

In the birthing room use essential oils in massage and hot compresses for pain relief. Cool compresses wiped on the forehead and face in between contractions will cool and relax, and add your chosen essential oils to a bowl of hot water or in a vaporizer to release soothing fragrances into the room.

Use about 8 drops of your chosen essential oils in a vaporizer to create the atmosphere you prefer for the room. Frankincense will help alleviate any fears, lavender will be calming and relaxing, and lemon and tea tree will freshen and disinfect the room. Clary sage and jasmine are effective in strengthening contractions. Jasmine may be cloying in the atmosphere of the birthing room so mix it with lavender and clary sage.

BIRTHING ROOM FRAGRANCES

bergamot 3 drops
lemon 3 drops
lavender 3 drops
This antibacterial blend has a light fragrance and will keep you alert. Sustitute geranium for lemon for second stage.

tea tree 4 drops
lavender 2 drops
lemon 2 drops
This antiseptic blend will purify the room.

frankincense 8 drops
This will slow and relax your breathing help disperse anxiety during the labor.

chamomile 4 drops
geranium 4 drops
This blend is calming.

neroli 3 drops
geranium 3 drops
ylang ylang 3 drops
For second stage.

Labor massage blends

These massage blends are for 2 oz (50 mls) of base oil.

Latent phase labor ("pre-labor"): frankincense
8 drops, sandalwood 3 drops, orange 2 drops, or
frankincense 15 drops.

First stage labor: lavender 15 drops; or lavender
7 drops, clary sage 5 drops, bergamot 3 drops.
Massage to lower back. Analgesic and calming and
balancing to the nervous system. Or try lavender
8 drops, rose or ylang ylang 7 drops.

Second stage labor: lavender 10 drops,
sandalwood or jasmine 5 drops: or clary sage 15 drops;
or clary sage 10 drops, rose 2 drops, ylang ylang 3 drops.
Try also inhaling 1 drop neroli or geranium on a tissue.

Third stage/After birth: rose 5 drops, clary sage
5 drops, geranium or frankincense 5 drops. A jasmine
massage will tone the uterine muscles.

Inhaling 1 drop neroli or lavender on a tissue will
help you relax and sleep after the birth.

For fear and anxiety during labor: lavender
10 drops and frankincense or sandalwood 5 drops.

Compresses for labor pain relief

Hot compress: clary sage 3 drops; or jasmine 1 drop,
lavender 1 drop, clary sage 1 drop. Good for first
stage. Use for lower abdomen or lower back pain and
if the thighs are in spasm. Replace as it cools.
Lavender and jasmine will strengthen contractions and
produce an analgesic effect. To help expel the placenta
try a compress with 3 drops lavender and jasmine.

Cold compress: lavender 2–3 drops on a cold
washcloth or in atomizer. Use on the face or forehead
to refresh. Good for second stage. Try rose or neroli or
lavender for transition stage.

A–Z

of postnatal health

Refer also to Healing Aromatics, page 39 and
Aromatherapy for Mind & Mood, page 27.

BREASTFEEDING

Vaporizer: 2 drops of either lemongrass, peppermint or fennel to promote breast milk

Bath: jasmine 2 drops, peppermint 2 drops

Use oils in very low doses on the breasts and if breastfeeding avoid direct contact with nipples or wash away any residue of essential oils before feeding. A cool compress with 1 drop each of lavender, geranium and eucalyptus or peppermint will help alleviate soreness. Add 1 drop each of rose, chamomile, lavender to 2 oz (50 mls) of sweet almond oil and use a half teaspoonful to gently massage the breasts.

Use warm compresses before breastfeeding and cold compresses after the feed. If the nipples are engorged, try geranium 10 drops and peppermint 5 drops in 2 oz (50 mls) base oil.

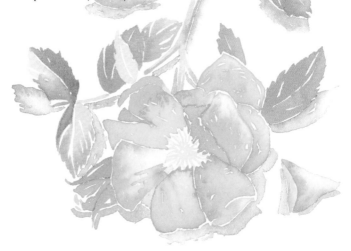

PERINEUM HEALING

Warm sitz bath: cypress 2 drops, lavender 3 drops

PERINEAL PAIN

Sitz bath: lavender 4 drops, tea tree 2 drops
Lavender and tea tree will also help heal tears and stitches.

POSTNATAL FATIGUE

Massage: bergamot 8 drops, geranium 8 drops, orange 4 drops, in 2 oz (50 mls) base carrier oil

Bath: geranium or bergamot 3 drops, rosemary 2 drops

Vaporizer: geranium 1 drop, lemon 2 drops

POSTNATAL DEPRESSION

Be kind to yourself during the "baby blues" and use essential oils to soothe and for a pick-me-up.

Uplifting: neroli, lemon, orange

Grounding: lavender, frankincense, sandalwood, patchouli

Use 2 drops from the uplifting oils and 1 drop of one of the grounding oils in the bath or in 2 teaspoons (10 mls) base oil.

Add your choice of the following blends to 2 oz (50 mls) base carrier oil for a massage, or to the bath if preferred:

1. Geranium 5 drops, clary sage 5 drops, lavender 10 drops
2. Neroli 8 drops, frankincense 6 drops, lemon or orange 2 drops
3. Bergamot 8 drops, clary sage 6 drops, rose 2 drops
4. Geranium 8 drops, frankincense 6 drops, jasmine 2 drops.

Babies and children

*Use very low dosages for babies and never
allow neat essential oils to touch their skin.
For children, use half or one-third
dosages recommended for adults.*

BABY SKIN RASH

Massage: Add 3 drops of lavender to 2 oz
(50 mls) sweet almond oil or jojoba oil.
Use a half teaspoonful and apply gently to the
baby's bottom.

BABY COLIC

Rub a little lavender in jojoba oil on your neck
before holding the baby to help get the baby
to sleep, or use lavender or chamomile in a
room vaporizer.

Add one drop of chamomile or lavender or
geranium to a glass bowl of warm water. Mix
and wring out a cotton cloth in the water and
apply the compress to the baby's stomach area.

BABY DRY SKIN

Add one drop of rose or chamomile or lavender
to 2 oz (50 mls) sweet almond oil or jojoba oil
and apply a little to baby's skin by stroking the
baby gently after bathing or changing.

Index

aching joints 40
acne 52, 55–8
aloe vera gel 41, 43, 49, 50
anger 28, 30
anise oil 69
antiseptic oils 26, 52
anxiety 28, 30–1
apathy 31
apricot kernel oil 10
aromabaths 19–22
arthritis 40
athlete's foot 40
atomizers 7, 14, 15–17, 57
avocado oil 10

babies and children 76
back pain 40
balancing oils 28, 29
base carrier oils 9, 10
base note oils 10
basil oil 11–12, 21, 24, 26, 28,
   30, 32–3, 37, 42–7, 49, 54, 68–9
bathroom freshener 24
baths 7, 19–22
beauty 51–62
bed linen perfumes 18
bergamot oil 11–12, 15–17, 20–1,
   24–6, 28–35, 37–8, 41–4, 46–7,
   49–50, 52–9, 62, 64–8, 70,
   72–3, 75
birthing room fragrances 72
bleeding cuts and wounds 40
blood pressure 40–1, 71
body massage base carrier oil
   blend 10
body massage blends 9, 53
boils 41
Braxton Hicks contractions 71

breastfeeding 74
bronchitis 41
bruises and sprains 41
burners *see* vaporizers
burns 41

camphor 52, 69
caraway oil 69
carrot oil 69
catarrh 41
cedarwood oil 11–12, 16, 18,
   20–2, 24–5, 28, 30, 34–5,
   37–8, 41, 43, 52–3, 60–2, 69
cellulite 42
chamomile oil 11–12, 20, 22, 28,
   30, 33–4, 36, 38, 41–2, 44–8,
   49–50, 52, 55, 57–61, 68–9,
   72, 74, 76
chilblains 42
children and babies 76
children's party fragrances 25
Christmas fragrances 25
cinnamon oil 69
citronella oil 24
clary sage oil 11–12, 17, 22, 24–5,
   28–9, 31–2, 38, 44, 47, 50, 57,
   60–1, 64, 66, 69, 72–3, 75
clay 56
cleansers, facial 57
clothing perfumes 18
clove oil 69
colds 42
colic, baby 76
cologne 14, 15
compresses 8, 55
concentration 28
confidence 28, 31
constipation 43

cramps 43, 47
cuts and wounds, bleeding 40
cypress oil 11–12, 20, 41–4,
   48–50, 52–6, 58–61, 69, 75
cystitis 43

dandruff 62
depression 28, 30–2, 35
dermatitis 43
despair 32
diarrhea 43
diffusers see vaporizers
direct application 8
disappointment 33

eau de toilette 14, 17
eczema 43
emotional exhaustion 33
eucalyptus oil 11–12, 20, 24, 33,
   37, 40–2, 46, 48–9, 52, 65, 62,
   68, 74
euphoria 28, 29
evening primrose oil 10, 71
exfoliation 59
exhaustion 44
eyes 44

facial base carrier oil blend 10
facial care 54–8
facial massage 54
fatigue 33
fear 28, 30
feet 7, 44, 48, 71
fennel oil 11–12, 20, 41–7, 55,
   58, 69, 74
footbaths 7
fragrancers see vaporizers
frankincense 11–12, 20–2, 24–5,
   28–31, 33–4, 36, 38, 43, 47,
   49, 52–4, 56, 58–9, 69–73, 75
'Fuller's Earth' 56

geranium oil 11–12, 15–18, 20–2,
   24–6, 28–30, 32–6, 38, 40–1,
   43–50, 52–9, 61–2, 64, 67–76
gout 44
grapefruit oil 11, 33, 37
grapeseed oil 10
grief 28, 34
grounding oils 29, 75
guilt 34

haemorrhoids 48–9
hair care 60–2
hand care 59
hangover 45
hazelnut oil 10
headache 45
   see also migraine
healing aromatics 39–50
heartburn see indigestion
high blood pressure 40, 71
hipbaths see sitz baths
hives 45
home and workplace fragrances
   23–6
housewarming fragrances 24
hyssop oil 11–12, 41–2, 52, 69

immune system 46
indigestion 46, 71
infections 46
influenza 46
inhalation 8
insect repellants 24
insomnia 22, 28, 35–6
irritability 28, 36
itchy scalp 62
itchy skin 52

jasmine oil 11–12, 16, 18, 28–31,
   33–4, 38, 44, 47, 52–3, 64–6,
   68–9, 72–5

relaxing baths 22
resentment 28
restorative oils 22, 29
revitalizing baths 22
room fresheners and fragrances 24, 66, 68
rose oil 11–12, 15–16, 18, 20–1, 25, 28–30, 32–6, 38, 40, 44–5, 47, 52–3, 55, 57–9, 61, 64–6, 68–71, 73–6
rosemary oil 11–12, 17, 20, 22, 26, 28, 32–3, 37, 40–50, 52–3, 59–62, 67–9, 75
rosewood oil 16–17, 25–6, 30, 33, 36, 44–5, 52–3, 58, 60–2, 64, 70

safflower oil 10
sage oil 47, 69
sandalwood oil 11–12, 16, 20, 24–5, 28–34, 37–8, 41–3, 46–8, 50, 52–5, 57–9, 61–2, 64–71, 73, 75
sassafras oil 69
sensual fragrances 63–6
showers 8
sinus 49
sitz baths 7
skin care 52–9
 baby 76
skin conditions 49
skin types 52–8
sprains and bruises 41
sprays *see* atomizers
spritzers *see* atomizers
St Valentine's Day fragrances 25

steaming, facial 55
stress 28, 38
stretch marks 71
sunburn 50
sunflower oil 10
sweet almond oil 10, 21, 54, 56, 59, 61, 71, 74, 76

tangerine oil 11, 69
tea tree oil 11–12, 24, 26, 40–3, 46, 49–50, 52–3, 56, 58, 62, 68, 72, 75
throat infections 50
thyme oil 11–12, 20, 40–1, 49, 52, 69
toners, facial 57
tonsillitis 50
top note oils 11
towels, perfumes for 18
travel 67–8

uplifting oils 29, 75

vaporizers 9
varicose veins 50
vitamin E oil 10, 56, 71

wheatgerm oil 10, 49, 71
witch hazel 58
workplace fragrances 26

ylang ylang oil 11–12, 16, 18, 20, 25, 28–33, 37, 40, 47, 52–3, 58, 64–6, 68, 70–3